OSTEOPOROSIS DIET COOKBOOK FOR SENIORS

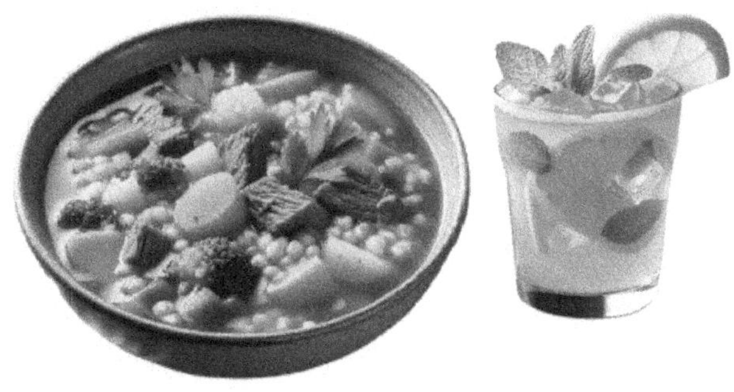

A Comprehensive Guide to a Nutrient-Rich Osteoporosis Diet

LANITA CRUZ

Copyright © 2024 by Lanita Cruz

TABLE OF CONTENT

Disclaimer

The information provided in this cookbook is for educational and informational purposes only. It is not intended to be a substitute for professional medical advice, diagnosis, or treatment.

Always seek the advice of your physician or other qualified health provider with any questions you may have regarding a medical condition.

The recipes and dietary suggestions included are based on general principles and may not be suitable for everyone.

Individual dietary needs and health conditions vary, and it is essential to consult with a healthcare professional before making significant changes to your diet.

The author and publisher disclaim responsibility for any effects resulting directly or indirectly from the use or misuse of the information provided in this cookbook.

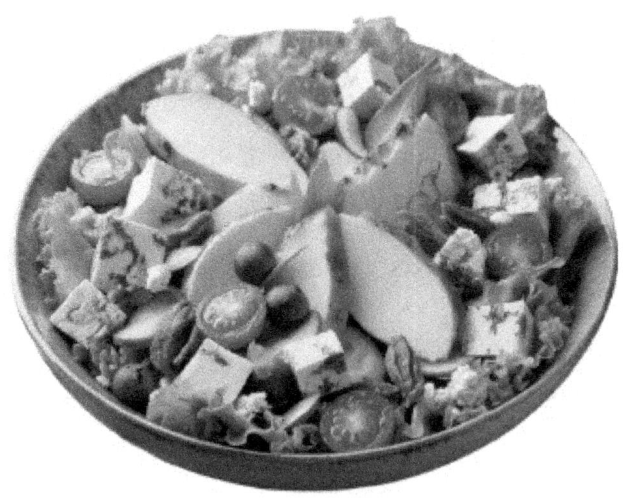

Introduction

Welcome to the "Osteoporosis Diet Cookbook for Seniors," a guide crafted with care to support the health and well-being of older individuals.

Osteoporosis causes the bones to become weak and brittle, making them more prone to fractures, it can have a significant impact on your quality of life, as it can limit your mobility, increase your pain, and reduce your independence.

However, osteoporosis is not inevitable. There are many ways to prevent and manage this condition, and one of the most important ones is diet.

Osteoporosis poses unique challenges, and nutrition plays a crucial role in managing its impact on bone health.

What you eat and drink can have a profound effect on your bone health, as it can provide the essential nutrients, such as calcium, vitamin D, protein, and magnesium that your bones need to be strong and healthy.

In this comprehensive cookbook, we delve into the principles of the osteoporosis diet, exploring the benefits it offers to seniors.

Whether you're seeking preventive measures or managing osteoporosis, this book provides valuable insights into foods to include and avoid, along with a handy shopping list.

Embark on a journey through nourishing recipes tailored for breakfast, lunch, and dinner, as well as delightful desserts and snacks.

Quench your thirst with specialized beverages, and let a 30-day meal plan guide you towards a balanced and bone-friendly diet.

Join us in prioritizing your health through informed choices and delectable meals.

CHAPTER 1

Principles of the Osteoporosis Diet

1. **Calcium-Rich Foods**: One fundamental principle of the osteoporosis diet is the emphasis on calcium-rich foods.

   Adequate calcium intake is crucial for maintaining bone density, and this section highlights dairy products, leafy greens, and fortified foods as excellent sources.

2. **Vitamin D Synergy**: Vitamin D works in tandem with calcium to promote bone health.

   This diet emphasizes foods rich in vitamin D, such as fatty fish, egg yolks, and fortified cereals, to ensure optimal calcium absorption and utilization.

3. **Protein Moderation:** While protein is essential for overall health, excessive intake, particularly from animal sources, may contribute to calcium loss.

   This diet recommends a balanced approach to protein, incorporating both plant-based and lean animal sources without overindulgence.

4. **Phosphorus Awareness:** Phosphorus is another mineral vital for bone health, but an imbalance with calcium can be detrimental.

   The diet is a guide to maintaining balance between these minerals, steering clear of excessive phosphorus-rich processed foods.

5. **Limiting Sodium Intake**: High sodium intake can lead to increased calcium excretion, potentially weakening bones.

   The osteoporosis diet encourages you to be mindful of your sodium intake, opting for fresh, whole foods over processed options.

6. **Magnesium Inclusion:** Magnesium plays a role in bone metabolism, and this diet promotes magnesium-rich foods like nuts, seeds, and whole grains.

   Ensuring an adequate magnesium intake complements the overall strategy for bone health.

7. **Balanced Nutrient Intake:** Beyond individual nutrients, the osteoporosis diet encourages a balanced and varied diet.

By including a range of nutrients from fruits, vegetables, whole grains, and lean proteins, you can support not only bone health but also overall well-being.

By understanding and incorporating these principles, you can proactively engage in a diet that supports bone health, reducing the risk and impact of osteoporosis.

Benefits of Osteoporosis Diet

1. **Enhanced Bone Density**: The foremost advantage of adopting an osteoporosis diet is the potential for enhanced bone density.

   This diet's focus on calcium, vitamin D, and other essential nutrients provides the foundation for maintaining and even improving bone strength.

2. **Fracture Prevention**: A well-balanced osteoporosis diet contributes to fracture prevention.

   By ensuring an adequate intake of nutrients crucial for bone health, you can reduce the risk of fractures, a common concern for individuals with osteoporosis.

3. **Improved Calcium Absorption**: The combination of calcium-rich foods and vitamin D in this diet promotes optimal calcium absorption. This synergy is essential for ensuring that the body effectively utilizes calcium for bone mineralization.

4. **Enhanced Muscle Function:** Beyond bone health, the osteoporosis diet benefits you by supporting overall musculoskeletal function. Adequate protein intake and a balanced nutrient profile contribute to muscle strength, aiding in mobility and reducing the risk of falls.

5. **Joint Health:** This diet's emphasis on a variety of nutrients, including omega-3 fatty acids and antioxidants from fruits and vegetables, supports joint health. This is particularly important as it helps mitigate discomfort and stiffness associated with aging.

6. **Maintained Weight and Body Composition**: Adopting a well-rounded osteoporosis diet can assist you in maintaining a healthy weight and body composition.

This, in turn, contributes to overall well-being and reduces the strain on bones and joints.

7. **Optimized Nutrient Intake**: By following the osteoporosis diet, you ensure they receive a well-rounded mix of essential nutrients.

   This helps address nutritional deficiencies that could otherwise impact bone health and overall vitality.

8. **Heart Health Benefits**: Some components of the osteoporosis diet, such as omega-3 fatty acids from fish, contribute to heart health.

   This dual benefit addresses cardiovascular concerns often associated with aging, promoting a holistic approach to well-being.

Foods to Eat

Dairy and Fortified Alternatives: Include low-fat dairy products like milk, yogurt, and cheese in your osteoporosis diet.

For those with lactose intolerance or opting for plant-based choices, fortified alternatives such as almond or soy milk can provide essential calcium and vitamin D.

Leafy Greens: Incorporate dark, leafy greens such as kale, spinach, and collard greens. These vegetables are rich in calcium, magnesium, and vitamin K, all contributing to bone health.

Fatty Fish: Integrate fatty fish like salmon, mackerel, and sardines into your diet. These sources are not only high in calcium but also provide omega-3 fatty acids, promoting overall cardiovascular and bone health.

Nuts and Seeds: Snack on nuts and seeds, such as almonds, chia seeds, and sunflower seeds. These are excellent sources of magnesium, which complements calcium absorption and supports bone metabolism.

Fortified Foods: Opt for foods fortified with calcium and vitamin D, such as fortified cereals, orange juice, and tofu. These additions ensure a consistent intake of these crucial nutrients, especially for those with dietary restrictions.

Lean Proteins: Protein is essential for muscle health, contributing to overall skeletal support and reducing the risk of falls, include lean protein sources like poultry, fish, beans, and legumes.

Whole Grains: Choose whole grains like brown rice, quinoa, and whole wheat bread, these grains provide a variety of nutrients, including magnesium and phosphorus, supporting bone health and overall well-being.

Fruits and Vegetables: Ensure a colorful array of fruits and vegetables in your diet.

These foods are rich in antioxidants, vitamins, and minerals that contribute to bone health and help combat oxidative stress.

Eggs: Incorporate eggs into your meals for a good source of vitamin D. Whether scrambled, boiled, or as part of a dish, eggs are a versatile addition to the osteoporosis diet.

Beans and Legumes: Beans and legumes, such as chickpeas and lentils, are excellent sources of protein, magnesium, and other minerals beneficial for bone health. Include them in salads, soups, or stews for a nutritious boost.

Foods to Avoid

Excessive Sodium Sources: Limit the intake of high-sodium foods, including processed and packaged items.

Excessive sodium can contribute to calcium loss, potentially weakening bones. Be mindful of canned soups, salty snacks, and ready-made meals.

Carbonated Beverages: Reduce consumption of carbonated beverages, as they may interfere with calcium absorption. The phosphoric acid in sodas can contribute to calcium depletion, impacting overall bone health.

High-Phosphorus Foods: Be cautious with foods high in phosphorus, as an imbalance with calcium can be detrimental.

Limit intake of processed meats, carbonated drinks, and certain processed foods that may contain phosphorus additives.

Caffeine-Heavy Products: Moderate your intake of caffeine-rich products, such as coffee and some teas. While moderate caffeine consumption is generally acceptable, excessive amounts can interfere with calcium absorption.

Alcohol in Excess: Limit alcohol consumption, as excessive alcohol intake can interfere with bone formation and increase the risk of fractures. Moderation is key to mitigating potential adverse effects on bone health.

High-Sugar Treats: Minimize the consumption of high-sugar treats, including candies, pastries, and sugary snacks.

Excessive sugar intake can negatively impact overall health, potentially contributing to inflammation and bone density issues.

Saturated and Trans Fats: Reduce the intake of saturated and trans fats, commonly found in fried foods and processed snacks.

These fats can compromise bone health and contribute to other health issues, including cardiovascular concerns.

Excessive Red Meat: While lean protein is essential, limit the intake of excessive red and processed meats. High consumption of these meats has been linked to increased bone loss and fracture risk.

High-Oxalate Foods: For those prone to kidney stones, limit high-oxalate foods like spinach, beets, and nuts, as they can interfere with calcium absorption. Adjust your diet under the guidance of a healthcare professional if necessary.

Refined and White Flour Products: Minimize the consumption of refined and white flour products, such as white bread and pastries, opt for whole grain alternatives to ensure a higher intake of beneficial nutrients for bone health.

Comprehensive Shopping List for Osteoporosis Diet

Dairy and Fortified Alternatives:

- Low-fat milk
- Yogurt (low-fat or Greek)
- Cheese (preferably low-fat or part-skim)
- Almond or soy milk (fortified with calcium and vitamin D)

Leafy Greens:

- Kale
- Spinach
- Collard greens

- Broccoli

Fatty Fish:

- Salmon

- Mackerel

- Sardines

Nuts and Seeds:

- Almonds

- Chia seeds

- Sunflower seeds

- Walnuts

Fortified Foods:

- Fortified cereals

- Fortified orange juice

- Tofu (fortified with calcium)

Lean Proteins:

- Skinless poultry (chicken or turkey)

- Fish (non-fatty varieties)

- Beans (kidney beans, black beans)

- Lentils

Whole Grains:

- Brown rice
- Quinoa
- Whole wheat bread
- Oats

Beans and Legumes:

- Chickpeas
- Lentils
- Black-eyed peas

Low-Sodium Seasonings:

- Herbs (such as basil, thyme, and oregano)
- Spices (like turmeric and cinnamon)

Low-Fat Dairy Alternatives:

- Greek yogurt (low-fat)
- Cottage cheese (low-fat)
- Almond or soy-based cheese

Lean Protein Sources:

- Skinless turkey or chicken breast

- Fish (salmon, trout)
- Legumes (beans, lentils)

Healthy Fats:

- Avocado
- Olive oil
- Flaxseeds

Whole Grains:

- Quinoa
- Brown rice
- Whole wheat pasta
- Oats

Vegetables:

- Broccoli
- Brussels sprouts
- Cauliflower
- Carrots
- Sweet potatoes

Fruits:

- Oranges

- Berries (blueberries, strawberries)

- Kiwi

- Pineapple

Nuts and Seeds:

- Almonds

- Walnuts

- Chia seeds

- Flaxseeds

Spices and Herbs:

- Turmeric

- Basil

- Thyme

- Oregano

CHAPTER 2

Breakfast Recipes for Osteoporosis Diet

Ricotta and Honey Toast

- **Preparation Time:** 5 minutes
- **Serves:** 1

Ingredients:

- 2 slices whole grain bread
- 1/2 cup ricotta cheese
- 1 tablespoon honey
- Fresh berries (optional, for garnish)

Nutritional Information: Calories: 320kcal, Protein: 15g, Carbohydrates: 35g, Fat: 15g, Fiber: 5g

Instructions:

1. Toast the whole grain bread slices until golden brown.
2. Spread a generous layer of ricotta cheese evenly on each slice.

3. Drizzle honey over the ricotta-covered toast.

4. Optionally, garnish with fresh berries for added flavor and nutritional benefits.

Serving Suggestions:

- Pair with a side of mixed berries or a cup of green tea for a well-balanced breakfast.

Greek Yogurt Parfait

- **Preparation Time:** 7 minutes
- **Serves:** 1

Ingredients:

- 1 cup Greek yogurt (low-fat)
- 1/2 cup granola (low-sugar)
- 1/2 cup mixed berries (strawberries, blueberries & raspberries)
- 1 tablespoon honey

Nutritional Information: Calories: 380kcal, Protein: 20g, Carbohydrates: 45g, Fat: 15g, Fiber: 6g

Instructions:

1. In a glass or bowl, layer half of the Greek yogurt at the bottom.
2. Add a layer of granola on top of the yogurt.
3. Place a portion of mixed berries over the granola.
4. Repeat the layers with the remaining yogurt, granola, and berries.
5. Drizzle honey over the top for a touch of sweetness.

Serving Suggestions:

- Serve chilled and enjoy as a wholesome and satisfying breakfast

Veggie and Hummus Wrap

- **Preparation Time:** 10 minutes
- **Serves:** 1

Ingredients:

- 1 whole wheat wrap
- 2 tablespoons hummus
- 1/2 cup mixed veggies (bell peppers, cucumber, cherry tomatoes)

- 1/4 cup baby spinach leaves
- Salt and pepper to taste

Nutritional Information: Calories: 280kcal, Protein: 10g, Carbohydrates: 40g, Fat: 10g, Fiber: 8g

Instructions:

1. Lay the whole wheat wrap on a clean surface.
2. Spread hummus evenly across the center of the wrap.
3. Place a layer of mixed veggies and baby spinach leaves over the hummus, season with salt and pepper to taste.
4. Tuck in the wrap's edges and make a firm roll.

Serving Suggestions:

- Slice the wrap in half and serve with a side of carrot sticks or a small green salad for a refreshing breakfast.

Whole Grain Waffles with Berry Compote

- **Preparation Time:** 15 minutes
- **Serves:** 2

Ingredients:

- 1 cup whole grain waffle mix
- 1 cup mixed berries (strawberries, blueberries & raspberries)
- 2 tablespoons honey
- Greek yogurt (low-fat) for topping

Nutritional Information: Calories: 320kcal per serving, Protein: 8g, Carbohydrates: 60g, Fat: 5g, Fiber: 6g

Instructions:

1. Prepare the whole grain waffle mix according to package instructions.
2. In a saucepan, heat the mixed berries and honey until they form a compote.
3. Cook the waffles until it turns golden brown and crisp.

4. Top the waffles with the berry compote.

5. Add a dollop of Greek yogurt on top.

Serving Suggestions:

- Serve warm, garnished with additional fresh berries and a sprinkle of chopped nuts for added texture and flavor.

Ham and Cheese Croissant

- **Preparation Time:** 12 minutes
- **Serves:** 1

Ingredients:

- 1 croissant (whole grain if available)

- 2 slices lean ham

- 1 slice Swiss cheese (low-fat)

- 1 teaspoon Dijon mustard

- Fresh lettuce leaves

Nutritional Information: Calories: 380kcal, Protein: 20g, Carbohydrates: 30g, Fat: 18g, Fiber: 2g

Instructions:

1. Preheat the oven and briefly warm the croissant.

2. Slice the croissant in half horizontally.

3. Spread Dijon mustard on the bottom half of the croissant.

4. Layer lean ham, Swiss cheese, and fresh lettuce leaves.

5. Place the top half of the croissant and press gently.

Serving Suggestions:

- Pair with a side of sliced melon or a small serving of mixed berries for a delightful and balanced breakfast.

Banana Oat Pancakes

- **Preparation Time:** 15 minutes

- **Serves:** 2

Ingredients:

- 1 cup rolled oats

- 1 ripe banana

- 2 eggs

- 1/2 cup Greek yogurt (low-fat)

- 1 teaspoon baking powder

- 1/2 teaspoon cinnamon
- Fresh berries for topping

Nutritional Information: Calories: 220kcal per serving, Protein: 12g, Carbohydrates: 30g, Fat: 6g, Fiber: 4g

Instructions:

1. In a blender, combine rolled oats, banana, eggs, Greek yogurt, baking powder, and cinnamon.
2. Blend until a smooth batter forms.
3. Heat a non-stick pan over medium heat and pour small portions of batter to form pancakes.
4. Cook the top side until bubbles show up, then switch to the bottom side and cook it.
5. Repeat until all the batter is used.

Serving Suggestions:

- Top the pancakes with a dollop of Greek yogurt and a handful of fresh berries for added flavor and nutritional benefits.

Tofu Scramble

- **Preparation Time:** 15 minutes
- **Serves:** 2

Ingredients:

- 1 tablespoon olive oil
- 1 block firm tofu, crumbled
- 1/2 cup diced bell peppers "assorted colors"
- 1/4 cup diced red onion
- 1 teaspoon turmeric
- Salt and pepper to taste
- Fresh herbs (parsley or chives) for garnish

Nutritional Information: Calories: 220kcal per serving, Protein: 15g, Carbohydrates: 10g, Fat: 14g, Fiber: 2g

Instructions:

1. Heat olive oil in a skillet over medium heat, add diced bell peppers and red onion, sauté until softened.
2. Crumble the tofu into the skillet, stirring gently.

3. Sprinkle turmeric over the tofu for color, season with salt and pepper to taste.

4. Continue cooking until the tofu is heated through.

Serving Suggestions:

- Serve the tofu scramble with a slice of whole grain toast or in a whole wheat wrap for a protein-packed and savory breakfast option.

Lunch Recipes for Osteoporosis Diet

Bison Burgers with Sweet Potato Fries

- **Preparation Time:** 30 minutes
- **Serves:** 4

Ingredients:

- 1 lb ground bison
- 1/2 teaspoon garlic powder
- 1/2 teaspoon onion powder
- Salt and pepper to taste
- 4 whole grain burger buns
- Toppings: Lettuce, tomato, red onion, pickles

Sweet Potato Fries:

- 2 large sweet potatoes, peeled and cut into fries
- 1 tablespoon olive oil
- 1 teaspoon paprika
- Salt and pepper to taste

Nutritional Information: Calories: 380kcal per serving, Protein: 27g, Carbohydrates: 38g, Fat: 14g, Fiber: 6g

Instructions:

1. Preheat the oven to 425°F (220°C).
2. In a bowl, mix the ground bison with garlic powder, onion powder, salt, and pepper. Shape into four burger patties.
3. Place sweet potato fries on a baking sheet. Drizzle with olive oil, sprinkle with paprika, salt, and pepper, toss to coat evenly.
4. Bake the sweet potato fries for 25-30 minutes or until crispy, turning once.
5. While fries are baking, grill bison burgers for about 4-5 minutes per side or until cooked to your preferred doneness.
6. Toast the whole grain burger buns on the grill for a minute.

7. Assemble burgers with lettuce, tomato slices, red onion, and pickles.

8. Serve Bison Burgers with Sweet Potato Fries.

Serving Suggestions:

- Pair with a side of Greek yogurt-based dipping sauce for the sweet potato fries and a crisp green salad for a wholesome and bone-friendly lunch.

Thick Frittata with Zucchini

- **Preparation Time:** 25 minutes
- **Serves:** 4

Ingredients:

- 6 large eggs
- 1 cup shredded zucchini
- 1/2 cup diced red bell pepper
- 1/4 cup diced red onion
- 1/2 cup feta cheese (low-fat)
- Salt and pepper to taste
- 1 tablespoon olive oil

Nutritional Information: Calories: 220kcal per serving, Protein: 15g, Carbohydrates: 6g, Fat: 16g, Fiber: 2g

Instructions:

1. Preheat the oven to 375°F (190°C).
2. In a bowl, whisk together eggs, shredded zucchini, diced red bell pepper, diced red onion, and feta cheese, season the mixture with salt and pepper to taste.
3. Heat olive oil in an oven-safe skillet over medium heat, pour the egg mixture into the skillet, spreading it evenly.
4. Cook on the stovetop for 3-4 minutes until the edges begin to set.
5. Transfer the skillet to the preheated oven and bake for 15-18 minutes until the frittata is cooked through and slightly golden.
6. Allow the frittata to cool for a few minutes before slicing.

Serving Suggestions:

- Serve the Thick Frittata with Zucchini slices alongside a mixed green salad or whole grain bread for a nutritious lunch.

Bean & Tuna Salad with White Balsamic Vinegar

- **Preparation Time:** 15 minutes
- **Serves:** 2

Ingredients:

- 1 can /15 oz cannellini beans, drained and rinsed
- 1 can /5 oz tuna, drained
- 1/2 cup cherry tomatoes, halved
- 1/4 cup red onion, finely chopped
- 2 tablespoons fresh parsley, chopped
- 1 tablespoon white balsamic vinegar
- 1 tablespoon olive oil
- Salt and pepper to taste

Nutritional Information: Calories: 280kcal per serving, Protein: 22g, Carbohydrates: 32g, Fat: 9g, Fiber: 9g

Instructions:

1. In a large bowl, combine cannellini beans, tuna, cherry tomatoes, red onion, and fresh parsley.
2. In a small bowl, whisk together white balsamic vinegar and olive oil.
3. Pour the dressing over the bean and tuna mixture.
4. Gently toss the ingredients until well combined, season with salt and pepper to taste.

Serving Suggestions:

- Serve the Bean and Tuna Salad with White Balsamic Vinegar over a bed of mixed greens or whole grain crackers for a light and protein-packed lunch.

Scrambled Eggs with Dates

- **Preparation Time:** 10 minutes
- **Serves:** 2

Ingredients:

- 4 large eggs

- 2 tablespoons milk (low-fat)

- 4 Medjool dates, pitted and chopped

- 1 tablespoon butter

- Salt and pepper to taste

- Fresh chives for garnish (optional)

Nutritional Information: Calories: 220kcal per serving, Protein: 12g, Carbohydrates: 20g, Fat: 11g, Fiber: 2g

Instructions:

1. Whisk eggs and milk together in a bowl, until it is well combined.

2. Heat butter in a non-stick skillet over medium heat, add chopped dates to the skillet and sauté for 1-2 minutes until slightly softened.

3. Pour the whisked eggs into the skillet with dates.

4. Continuously stir the eggs until they are scrambled and cooked to your liking.

5. Season with salt and pepper to taste, garnish with fresh chives if desired.

Serving Suggestions:

- Serve the Scrambled Eggs with Dates on whole grain toast or alongside a side of fresh fruit for a sweet and savory lunch.

Turkey-Roquefort Salad

- **Preparation Time:** 20 minutes
- **Serves:** 2

Ingredients:

- 2 cups mixed salad greens
- 1 cup cooked turkey breast, sliced
- 1/4 cup Roquefort or blue cheese, crumbled
- 1/2 cup cherry tomatoes, halved
- 1/4 cup walnuts, toasted
- 2 tablespoons balsamic vinaigrette dressing

Nutritional Information: Calories: 280kcal per serving, Protein: 20g, Carbohydrates: 10g, Fat: 18g, Fiber: 4g

Instructions:

1. In a large bowl, combine mixed salad greens, sliced turkey breast, crumbled Roquefort cheese, cherry tomatoes, and toasted walnuts.

2. Drizzle the balsamic vinaigrette dressing over the salad and toss gently until the ingredients are well coated with the dressing.

3. Serve immediately.

Serving Suggestions:

- Pair the Turkey-Roquefort Salad with a side of whole grain bread or a cup of vegetable soup for a satisfying and protein-rich lunch.

Grilled Pesto Pizza

- **Preparation Time:** 30 minutes
- **Serves:** 2

Ingredients:

- 2 whole grain pizza crusts
- 1/2 cup basil pesto
- 1 cup cherry tomatoes, sliced
- 1/2 cup baby spinach leaves
- 1/2 cup mozzarella cheese, shredded (low-fat)
- 1 tablespoon pine nuts, toasted

Nutritional Information: Calories: 350kcal per serving, Protein: 15g, Carbohydrates: 45g, Fat: 14g, Fiber: 5g

Instructions:

1. Preheat the grill or oven to 400°F (200°C).
2. Place the whole grain pizza crusts on the grill or in the oven for a few minutes until they start to crisp.
3. Spread basil pesto evenly over the crusts.
4. Arrange sliced cherry tomatoes and baby spinach leaves on top.
5. Sprinkle shredded mozzarella cheese over the vegetables.
6. Grill or bake the pizzas until the cheese is melted and bubbly.
7. Remove from heat and sprinkle with toasted pine nuts.

Serving Suggestions:

- Slice the Grilled Pesto Pizza into wedges and serve with a side salad of mixed greens for a delightful and osteoporosis-friendly lunch.

Chicken and Vegetable Stir-Fry

- **Preparation Time:** 20 minutes
- **Serves:** 4

Ingredients:

- 1 lb boneless, skinless chicken breast, thinly sliced
- 2 tablespoons soy sauce (low-sodium)
- 1 tablespoon oyster sauce
- 1 tablespoon cornstarch
- 2 tablespoons vegetable oil
- 1 bell pepper, thinly sliced
- 1 cup broccoli florets
- 1 carrot, julienned
- 2 cloves garlic, minced
- 1 teaspoon fresh ginger, grated
- 2 green onions, sliced
- Sesame seeds for garnish (optional)

Nutritional Information: Calories: 280kcal per serving, Protein: 25g, Carbohydrates: 12g, Fat: 15g, Fiber: 3g

Instructions:

1. In a bowl, mix soy sauce, oyster sauce, and cornstarch to create a marinade. Add sliced chicken and let it marinate for 10 minutes.

2. Heat vegetable oil in a wok or large skillet over medium-high heat, add marinated chicken to the wok and stir-fry until fully cooked, remove chicken from the wok and set aside.

3. In the same wok, add a bit more oil if needed, stir-fry garlic and ginger until fragrant.

4. Add bell pepper, broccoli, and julienned carrot. Stir-fry for 3-4 minutes until vegetables are crisp-tender.

5. Return the cooked chicken to the wok and toss everything together until well combined.

6. Sprinkle sliced green onions over the stir-fry and toss for an additional minute.

7. Garnish with sesame seeds if desired.

Serving Suggestions:

- Serve the Chicken and Vegetable Stir-Fry over brown rice or quinoa for a balanced and nutritious meal.

Dinner Recipes for Osteoporosis Diet

Cod with Tomatoes and Black Olives

- **Preparation Time:** 25 minutes
- **Serves:** 4

Ingredients:

- 4 cod fillets (6 oz each)
- Salt and pepper to taste
- 2 tablespoons olive oil
- 1 onion, finely chopped
- 2 cloves garlic, minced
- 1 can /14 oz diced tomatoes, drained
- 1/2 cup black olives, sliced
- 1 teaspoon dried oregano
- 1/2 teaspoon red pepper flakes (optional)
- Fresh basil leaves for garnish

Nutritional Information: Calories: 280kcal per serving, Protein: 30g, Carbohydrates: 8g, Fat: 14g, Fiber: 3g

Instructions:

1. Preheat the oven to 400°F (200°C), season the cod fillets with salt and pepper on both sides.

2. In an ovenproof skillet, heat olive oil over medium heat, sear the cod fillets for 2-3 minutes on each side until golden brown, remove from the skillet and set aside.

3. Sauté chopped onion and minced garlic in the same skillet, until softened.

4. Add diced tomatoes, sliced black olives, dried oregano, and red pepper flakes (if using). Cook for 5 minutes.

5. Place the seared cod fillets on top of the tomato and olive mixture.

6. Transfer the skillet to the preheated oven and bake for 10-12 minutes or until the cod is cooked through.

7. Decorate with fresh basil leaves before serving.

Serving Suggestions:

- Serve the Cod with Tomatoes and Black Olives over a bed of quinoa or couscous and steamed vegetables for a Mediterranean-inspired dinner.

Veal Cordon Bleu

- **Preparation Time:** 30 minutes
- **Serves:** 4

Ingredients:

- 4 veal cutlets (4 oz each)
- Salt and pepper to taste
- 4 slices Swiss cheese (low-fat)
- 4 slices lean ham
- 1/2 cup whole wheat breadcrumbs
- 2 tablespoons olive oil
- 1 tablespoon Dijon mustard
- Fresh parsley for garnish

Nutritional Information: Calories: 320kcal per serving, Protein: 28g, Carbohydrates: 12g, Fat: 16g, Fiber: 2g

Instructions:

1. Preheat the oven to 375°F (190°C), season veal cutlets with salt and pepper.
2. Place a slice of Swiss cheese and a slice of lean ham on each veal cutlet.
3. Roll up the veal, securing the ends with toothpicks.

4. Spread Dijon mustard over the veal rolls.

5. Roll the veal in whole wheat breadcrumbs, ensuring an even coating.

6. In an ovenproof skillet, heat olive oil over medium heat.

7. Sear the veal rolls until golden brown on all sides.

8. Transfer the skillet to the preheated oven and bake for 15-18 minutes until veal is cooked through.

9. Garnish with fresh parsley before serving.

Serving Suggestions: Serve Veal Cordon Bleu with a side of steamed green beans or a mixed green salad for a classic and flavorful dinner.

Gingered Salmon Croquettes

- **Preparation Time:** 20 minutes

- **Serves:** 4

Ingredients:

- 2 cans (14 oz each) pink salmon, drained and flaked

- 1/2 cup whole wheat breadcrumbs

- 2 green onions, finely chopped

- 1 tablespoon fresh ginger, grated

- 1 tablespoon low-sodium soy sauce

- 1 tablespoon olive oil

- 1 egg, beaten

- Salt and pepper to taste

- Lemon wedges for serving

Nutritional Information: Calories: 240kcal per serving, Protein: 28g, Carbohydrates: 10g, Fat: 10g, Fiber: 2g

Instructions:

1. In a bowl, combine pink salmon, whole wheat breadcrumbs, chopped green onions, grated fresh ginger, soy sauce, and beaten egg.
2. Mix the ingredients until well combined.
3. Form the mixture into salmon patties.
4. Heat olive oil in a skillet over medium heat.
5. Cook the salmon patties for 3-4 minutes on each side until golden brown.
6. Season with salt and pepper to taste, serve with lemon wedges on the side.

Serving Suggestions:

- Enjoy Gingered Salmon Croquettes with a side of quinoa or brown rice and steamed broccoli for a nutritious and omega-3 rich dinner.

Beetroot Soup with Prune Dumplings

- **Preparation Time:** 40 minutes
- **Serves:** 4

Ingredients:

- 4 medium-sized beetroots, peeled and diced
- 1 onion, chopped
- 2 carrots, peeled and sliced
- 2 cloves garlic, minced
- 4 cups vegetable broth (low-sodium)
- 1 teaspoon caraway seeds
- Salt and pepper to taste
- 1 cup prunes, pitted and chopped
- 1 cup whole wheat breadcrumbs

- 1 egg, beaten
- Fresh dill for garnish

Nutritional Information: Calories: 180kcal per serving, Protein: 5g, Carbohydrates: 40g, Fat: 2g, Fiber: 7g

Instructions:

1. In a large pot, sauté chopped onions and minced garlic until translucent.
2. Add diced beetroots and sliced carrots to the pot. Cook for 5 minutes.
3. Pour in the vegetable broth, add caraway seeds, salt, and pepper, bring to a boil, then reduce heat and simmer until vegetables are tender.
4. In a bowl, combine chopped prunes, whole wheat breadcrumbs, and beaten egg to form a dough.
5. Shape the dough into small dumplings.
6. Drop the dumplings into the simmering soup, cook for an additional 10-12 minutes.
7. Garnish with fresh dill before serving.

Serving Suggestions:

- Serve Beetroot Soup with Prune Dumplings alongside a slice of whole grain bread or a light salad for a unique and healthy dinner option.

Picadillo

- **Preparation Time:** 35 minutes
- **Serves:** 4

Ingredients:

- 1 lb lean ground beef
- 1 onion, finely chopped
- 2 cloves garlic, minced
- 1 bell pepper, diced
- 14 oz (1 can) diced tomatoes, undrained
- 1/2 cup raisins
- 1/4 cup green olives, sliced
- 2 teaspoons ground cumin
- 1 teaspoon ground cinnamon
- Salt and pepper to taste

- 1/4 cup fresh cilantro, chopped
- Cooked brown rice for serving

Nutritional Information: Calories: 320kcal per serving, Protein: 25g, Carbohydrates: 30g, Fat: 12g, Fiber: 5g

Instructions:

1. In a large skillet, brown lean ground beef over medium heat, add chopped onions and minced garlic to the skillet. Cook until onions are softened.
2. Stir in diced bell peppers and cook for extra 3-4 minutes.
3. Add diced tomatoes, raisins, sliced green olives, ground cumin, ground cinnamon, salt, and pepper, simmer for 15-20 minutes.
4. Adjust seasoning if necessary and stir in fresh cilantro before serving.
5. Serve Picadillo over cooked brown rice.

Serving Suggestions:

- Pair Picadillo with a side of black beans or a mixed green salad for a flavorful and satisfying dinner.

Quiche Lorraine

- **Preparation Time:** 45 minutes
- **Serves:** 6

Ingredients:

- 1 pre-made whole grain pie crust
- 1 cup lean ham, diced
- 1 cup Swiss cheese, shredded
- 1/2 cup onion, finely chopped
- 4 large eggs
- 1 1/2 cups low-fat milk
- 1/4 teaspoon ground nutmeg
- Salt and pepper to taste
- Fresh chives for garnish

Nutritional Information: Calories: 280kcal per serving, Protein: 20g, Carbohydrates: 18g, Fat: 14g, Fiber: 2g

Instructions:

1. Preheat the oven to 375°F (190°C).

2. Place the whole grain pie crust in a pie dish and set aside.

3. In a bowl, mix diced lean ham, shredded Swiss cheese, and chopped onions, spread this mixture evenly over the pie crust.

4. In another bowl, whisk together eggs, low-fat milk, ground nutmeg, salt, and pepper.

5. Pour the egg mixture over the ham, cheese, and onion in the pie crust.

6. Bake in the preheated oven for 30-35 minutes or until the quiche is set and lightly browned.

7. Allow the quiche to cool for a few minutes before slicing.

8. Garnish with fresh chives before serving.

Serving Suggestions:

- Serve Quiche Lorraine with a side of mixed greens or a light soup for a delightful and protein-packed dinner.

Asparagus Gratin with Spring Leeks

- **Preparation Time:** 30 minutes
- **Serves:** 4

Ingredients:

- 1 lb asparagus, trimmed
- 2 leeks, thinly sliced, (the white & light green parts only)
- 2 tablespoons olive oil
- 2 tablespoons whole wheat flour
- 1 1/2 cups low-fat milk
- 1 cup Gruyere cheese, shredded
- Salt and pepper to taste
- 1/4 cup breadcrumbs
- Fresh parsley for garnish

Nutritional Information: Calories: 220kcal per serving, Protein: 12g, Carbohydrates: 18g, Fat: 12g, Fiber: 5g

Instructions:

1. Preheat the oven to 400°F (200°C).

2. Bring a pot of salted water to boil, blanch asparagus for 2 minutes, then transfer to an ice bath to stop the cooking process. Drain and set aside.

3. In a skillet, sauté thinly sliced leeks in olive oil until softened.

4. Sprinkle whole wheat flour over the leeks and stir to combine.

5. Slowly pour in low-fat milk, stirring constantly until the mixture thickens.

6. Stir in shredded Gruyere cheese until melted and smooth. Season with salt and pepper.

7. Arrange blanched asparagus in a baking dish. Pour the cheese and leek mixture over the asparagus.

8. In a small bowl, mix breadcrumbs with a bit of olive oil. Sprinkle over the asparagus.

9. Bake in the preheated oven for 15-18 minutes or until the top is golden brown.

10. Garnish with fresh parsley before serving.

Serving Suggestions:

- Serve Asparagus Gratin with Spring Leeks alongside grilled chicken or fish for a flavorful and nutritious dinner.

Desserts and Snacks for Osteoporosis Diet

Almond Stuffed Prunes in Chocolate

- **Preparation Time:** 20 minutes
- **Serves:** 12

Ingredients:

- 24 large prunes, pitted
- 24 almonds, blanched
- 8 oz dark chocolate, chopped
- 1 tablespoon coconut oil
- 1/4 cup shredded coconut (optional)

Nutritional Information: Calories: 120kcal per serving, Protein: 2g, Carbohydrates: 12g, Fat: 8g, Fiber: 2g

Instructions:

1. Gently slit each prune and insert a blanched almond inside, closing the prune around it.
2. In a heatproof bowl, melt the dark chocolate and coconut oil together, either in a microwave or using a double boiler.

3. Dip each stuffed prune into the melted chocolate, ensuring it's evenly coated.

4. Place the coated prunes on a parchment-lined tray and refrigerate until the chocolate sets.

5. Optionally, sprinkle shredded coconut over the chocolate before it sets.

6. Once set, transfer the prunes to an airtight container and store in the refrigerator.

Serving Suggestions:

- Serve Almond Stuffed Prunes in Chocolate as a sweet treat on their own or as a delightful addition to a dessert platter.

Red Marvel Smoothie

- **Preparation Time:** 10 minutes
- **Serves:** 2

Ingredients:

- 1 cup frozen mixed berries (strawberries, raspberries & blueberries)
- 1 medium-sized beetroot, peeled and diced
- 1 medium-sized carrot, peeled and sliced

- 1 cup unsweetened almond milk
- 1 tablespoon chia seeds
- 1 tablespoon honey (optional)
- Ice cubes (optional)

Nutritional Information: Calories: 120kcal per serving, Protein: 3g, Carbohydrates: 22g, Fat: 3g, Fiber: 6g

Instructions:

1. In a blender, combine frozen mixed berries, diced beetroot, sliced carrot, almond milk, and chia seeds.
2. Blend until smooth and creamy.
3. Taste and add honey if additional sweetness is desired.
4. If a colder consistency is preferred, add ice cubes and blend again until smooth, pour the smoothie into glasses and serve immediately.

Serving Suggestions:

- Enjoy the Red Marvel Smoothie as a refreshing and nutrient-packed snack between meals.

Raspberry Lemon Cake

- **Preparation Time:** 40 minutes
- **Serves:** 8

Ingredients:

- 1 1/2 cups whole wheat flour
- 1 1/2 teaspoons baking powder
- 1/4 teaspoon salt
- 1/2 cup unsalted butter, softened
- 1 cup granulated sugar
- 2 large eggs
- 1 teaspoon vanilla extract
- 1/2 cup Greek yogurt
- Zest of 1 lemon
- 1 1/2 cups fresh raspberries

Nutritional Information: Calories: 280kcal per serving, Protein: 5g, Carbohydrates: 40g, Fat: 12g, Fiber: 3g

Instructions:

1. Preheat the oven to 350°F (175°C). Grease and flour a cake pan.

2. In a bowl, whisk together whole wheat flour, baking powder, and salt.

3. In a separate large bowl, cream together softened butter and granulated sugar until light and fluffy.

4. Beat in eggs one at a time, then stir in vanilla extract.

5. Gradually mix in the dry ingredients, alternating with Greek yogurt.

6. Fold in lemon zest and gently stir in fresh raspberries.

7. Pour the batter into the prepared cake pan, spreading it evenly.

8. Bake in the preheated oven for 32-35 minutes or until a toothpick inserted into the center comes out clean.

9. Allow the cake to cool before slicing.

Serving Suggestions:

*   Serve Raspberry Lemon Cake with a dollop of Greek yogurt or a dusting of powdered sugar for a delightful dessert or afternoon treat.

Mini Pineapple Muffins

- **Preparation Time:** 25 minutes
- **Serves:** 12

Ingredients:

- 1 cup whole wheat flour
- 1/2 cup rolled oats
- 1 teaspoon baking powder
- 1/2 teaspoon baking soda
- 1/4 teaspoon salt
- 1/4 cup coconut oil, melted
- 1/3 cup honey
- 1 large egg
- 1 teaspoon vanilla extract
- 1/2 cup Greek yogurt
- 1/2 cup crushed pineapple, drained
- 1/4 cup shredded coconut (optional)

Nutritional Information: Calories: 140kcal per serving, Protein: 3g, Carbohydrates: 20g, Fat: 6g, Fiber: 2g

Instructions:

1. Preheat the oven to 350°F (175°C). Grease a mini muffin tin.
2. In a bowl, combine whole wheat flour, rolled oats, baking powder, baking soda, and salt.
3. In another bowl, whisk together melted coconut oil, honey, egg, vanilla extract, and Greek yogurt.
4. Add the wet ingredients to the dry one and mix until it is just combined.
5. Fold in crushed pineapple.
6. Spoon the batter into the mini muffin tin, filling each cup about 2/3 full.
7. If desired, sprinkle shredded coconut on top of each muffin.
8. Bake in the preheated oven for 12-15 minutes or until a toothpick inserted into the center comes out clean, allow the muffins to cool before serving.

Serving Suggestions:

- Enjoy Mini Pineapple Muffins as a bite-sized snack.

Black Bean Brownies

- **Preparation Time:** 30 minutes
- **Serves:** 16

Ingredients:

- 15 oz /1 can black beans, drained & rinsed
- 3 large eggs
- 1/3 cup coconut oil, melted
- 1/4 cup unsweetened cocoa powder
- 1/8 teaspoon salt
- 2 teaspoons vanilla extract
- 1/2 cup honey or maple syrup
- 1/2 cup whole wheat flour
- 1/2 cup dark chocolate chips

Nutritional Information: Calories: 120kcal per serving, Protein: 3g, Carbohydrates: 15g, Fat: 6g, Fiber: 3g

Instructions:

1. Preheat the oven to 350°F (175°C). Grease a baking pan.
2. In a food processor, blend black beans until smooth.

3. Add eggs, melted coconut oil, cocoa powder, salt, vanilla extract, and honey (or maple syrup) to the black bean puree. Blend until well combined.

4. Add whole wheat flour and blend again until smooth.

5. Fold in dark chocolate chips.

6. Pour the batter into the greased baking pan, spreading it evenly.

7. Bake in the preheated oven for 20-25 minutes or until a toothpick inserted into the center comes out with moist crumbs.

8. Allow the brownies to cool down before cutting it into squares.

Serving Suggestions:

- Serve Black Bean Brownies with a dollop of Greek yogurt or a sprinkle of chopped nuts for a healthier twist on a classic dessert.

Beverages/Drinks for Osteoporosis Diet

Prune and Pineapple Juice

- **Preparation Time:** 15 minutes
- **Serves:** 2

Ingredients:

- 1 cup pitted prunes
- 1 cup fresh pineapple chunks
- 1 tablespoon honey (optional)
- 2 cups water
- Ice cubes (optional)
- Mint leaves for garnish

Nutritional Information: Calories: 140kcal per serving, Protein: 2g, Carbohydrates: 36g, Fat: 0g, Fiber: 4g

Instructions:

1. In a blender, combine pitted prunes, fresh pineapple chunks, and water.
2. Blend until smooth.
3. Strain the mixture to remove pulp if desired.

4. If you prefer a sweeter taste, add honey and stir until dissolved.

5. Refrigerate the juice until chilled.

6. Serve over ice cubes and garnish with fresh mint leaves.

Serving Suggestions:

- Prune and Pineapple Juice is a delicious and fiber-rich beverage. Enjoy it as a refreshing morning drink or as a mid-afternoon pick-me-up.

Kefir

- **Preparation Time:** 5 minutes (plus fermentation time)
- **Serves:** Varies

Ingredients:

- 1 cup kefir grains
- 4 cups whole milk (preferably organic)
- 1 tablespoon honey (optional)

Nutritional Information: Varies based on fermentation time and type of milk used

Instructions:

1. Place kefir grains in a clean glass jar.
2. Pour whole milk over the kefir grains, leaving some space at the top of the jar.
3. If desired, add honey for sweetness.
4. Stir the mixture gently with a non-metal spoon.
5. Cover the jar with a clean cloth or paper towel and secure it with a rubber band.
6. Allow the mixture to ferment at room temperature for 12-48 hours. The longer the fermentation, the thicker and tangier the kefir.
7. After fermentation, strain the kefir to separate the grains. Use a plastic or wooden strainer; avoid metal.
8. Transfer the strained kefir to a clean jar for storage in the refrigerator.
9. Keep the kefir grains to reuse for the next batch.

Serving Suggestions:

- Enjoy Kefir on its own or blend it with fresh fruits for a delicious smoothie.

Grapefruit Juice

- **Preparation Time:** 10 minutes
- **Serves:** 2

Ingredients:

- 2 large grapefruits
- 1 tablespoon honey (optional)
- Ice cubes (optional)

Nutritional Information: Calories: 50kcal per serving, Protein: 1g, Carbohydrates: 13g, Fat: 0g, Fiber: 2g

Instructions:

1. Cut the grapefruits in half.
2. Using a citrus juicer, extract the juice from each grapefruit half.
3. Strain the juice to remove pulp and seeds if desired.
4. If you prefer a sweeter taste, add honey and stir until dissolved.
5. Refrigerate the juice until chilled.
6. Serve over ice cubes if you like it cold.

Serving Suggestions:

- Enjoy Grapefruit Juice as a refreshing beverage in the morning or as a thirst-quenching option throughout the day.

Fortified Alt-Milks

- **Preparation Time:** 10 minutes
- **Serves:** Varies

Ingredients:

- 4 cups unsweetened fortified plant-based milk (e.g., almond, soy, oat)
- 1 tablespoon maple syrup (optional)
- 1 teaspoon vanilla extract (optional)

Nutritional Information: Varies based on the type of plant-based milk used

Instructions:

1. In a saucepan, heat the plant-based milk over medium heat until warm but not boiling.
2. Add maple syrup and vanilla extract for sweetness and flavor, if desired.

3. Stir the mixture until well combined, remove from heat and let it cool slightly.

4. Pour the fortified alt-milk into a clean bottle or jar for storage, store in the refrigerator and shake well before serving.

Serving Suggestions:

- Fortified Alt-Milks can be used in coffee, tea, cereals, or enjoyed on their own. Use them as a dairy-free alternative in recipes that call for milk.

Mixed Berry Juice

- **Preparation Time:** 15 minutes
- **Serves:** 2

Ingredients:

- 1 cup strawberries, hulled
- 1/2 cup blueberries
- 1/2 cup raspberries
- 1 tablespoon honey (optional)
- 1 cup water
- Ice cubes (optional)
- Fresh mint leaves for garnish

Nutritional Information: Calories: 60kcal per serving, Protein: 1g, Carbohydrates: 15g, Fat: 0g, Fiber: 4g

Instructions:

1. Rinse the berries thoroughly.
2. In a blender, combine strawberries, blueberries, raspberries, and water.
3. Blend until smooth.
4. Strain the mixture to remove seeds and pulp if desired.
5. If you prefer a sweeter taste, add honey and stir until dissolved.
6. Refrigerate the juice until chilled.
7. Serve over ice cubes and garnish with fresh mint leaves.

Serving Suggestions:

- Mixed Berry Juice is a delightful and vitamin-rich beverage. Enjoy it on its own or mix it with sparkling water for a fizzy treat.

CHAPTER 3

30 Days Meal Plan for Osteoporosis Diet

Please note that the provided meal plan is a sample and should not be interpreted as a recommendation to consume all the listed recipes in a single day.

This meal plan aims to offer inspiration and guidance for healthy meal preparation. Feel free to customize this plan to suit your preferences and dietary requirements.

Day 1:

- **Breakfast:** Ricotta and Honey Toast
- **Lunch:** Bison Burgers with Sweet Potato Fries
- **Dinner:** Cod with Tomatoes and Black Olives
- **Snack:** Almond Stuffed Prunes in Chocolate

Day 2:

- **Breakfast:** Greek Yogurt Parfait
- **Lunch:** Thick Frittata with Zucchini
- **Dinner:** Veal Cordon Bleu

- **Snack:** Red Marvel Smoothie

Day 3:

- **Breakfast:** Veggie And Hummus Wrap
- **Lunch:** Bean and Tuna Salad with White Balsamic Vinegar
- **Dinner:** Gingered Salmon Croquettes
- **Snack:** Raspberry Lemon Cake

Day 4:

- **Breakfast:** Whole Grain Waffles with Berry Compote
- **Lunch:** Scrambled Eggs with Dates
- **Dinner:** Beetroot Soup with Prune Dumplings
- **Snack:** Mini Pineapple Muffins

Day 5:

- **Breakfast:** Ham and Cheese Croissant
- **Lunch:** Turkey-Roquefort Salad
- **Dinner:** Picadillo
- **Snack:** Black Bean Brownies

Day 6:

- **Breakfast:** Banana Oat Pancakes
- **Lunch:** Grilled Pesto Pizza
- **Dinner:** Quiche Lorraine
- **Snack:** Almond Stuffed Prunes in Chocolate

Day 7:

- **Breakfast:** Tofu Scramble
- **Lunch:** Chicken and Vegetable Stir-Fry
- **Dinner:** Asparagus Gratin with Spring Leeks
- **Snack:** Red Marvel Smoothie

Day 8:

- **Breakfast:** Ricotta and Honey Toast
- **Lunch:** Bison Burgers with Sweet Potato Fries
- **Dinner:** Cod with Tomatoes and Black Olives
- **Snack:** Raspberry Lemon Cake

Day 9:

- **Breakfast:** Greek Yogurt Parfait
- **Lunch:** Thick Frittata with Zucchini
- **Dinner:** Veal Cordon Bleu

- **Snack:** Mini Pineapple Muffins

Day 10:

- **Breakfast:** Veggie And Hummus Wrap
- **Lunch:** Bean and Tuna Salad with White Balsamic Vinegar
- **Dinner:** Gingered Salmon Croquettes
- **Snack:** Black Bean Brownies

Day 11:

- **Breakfast:** Whole Grain Waffles with Berry Compote
- **Lunch:** Scrambled Eggs with Dates
- **Dinner:** Beetroot Soup with Prune Dumplings
- **Snack:** Red Marvel Smoothie

Day 12:

- **Breakfast:** Ham and Cheese Croissant
- **Lunch:** Turkey-Roquefort Salad
- **Dinner:** Picadillo
- **Snack:** Almond Stuffed Prunes in Chocolate

Day 13:

- **Breakfast:** Banana Oat Pancakes
- **Lunch:** Grilled Pesto Pizza
- **Dinner:** Quiche Lorraine
- **Snack:** Raspberry Lemon Cake

Day 14:

- **Breakfast:** Tofu Scramble
- **Lunch:** Chicken and Vegetable Stir-Fry
- **Dinner:** Asparagus Gratin with Spring Leeks
- **Snack:** Mini Pineapple Muffins

Day 15:

- **Breakfast:** Ricotta and Honey Toast
- **Lunch:** Bison Burgers with Sweet Potato Fries
- **Dinner:** Cod with Tomatoes and Black Olives
- **Snack:** Black Bean Brownies

Day 16:

- **Breakfast:** Greek Yogurt Parfait
- **Lunch:** Thick Frittata with Zucchini
- **Dinner:** Veal Cordon Bleu

- **Snack:** Red Marvel Smoothie

Day 17:

- **Breakfast:** Veggie And Hummus Wrap
- **Lunch:** Bean and Tuna Salad with White Balsamic Vinegar
- **Dinner:** Gingered Salmon Croquettes
- **Snack:** Raspberry Lemon Cake

Day 18:

- **Breakfast:** Whole Grain Waffles with Berry Compote
- **Lunch:** Scrambled Eggs with Dates
- **Dinner:** Beetroot Soup with Prune Dumplings
- **Snack:** Mini Pineapple Muffins

Day 19:

- **Breakfast:** Ham and Cheese Croissant
- **Lunch:** Turkey-Roquefort Salad
- **Dinner:** Picadillo
- **Snack:** Black Bean Brownies

Day 20:

- **Breakfast:** Banana Oat Pancakes
- **Lunch:** Grilled Pesto Pizza
- **Dinner:** Quiche Lorraine
- **Snack:** Almond Stuffed Prunes in Chocolate

Day 21:

- **Breakfast:** Tofu Scramble
- **Lunch:** Chicken and Vegetable Stir-Fry
- **Dinner:** Asparagus Gratin with Spring Leeks
- **Snack:** Red Marvel Smoothie

Day 22:

- **Breakfast:** Ricotta and Honey Toast
- **Lunch:** Bison Burgers with Sweet Potato Fries
- **Dinner:** Cod with Tomatoes and Black Olives
- **Snack:** Raspberry Lemon Cake

Day 23:

- **Breakfast:** Greek Yogurt Parfait
- **Lunch:** Thick Frittata with Zucchini
- **Dinner:** Veal Cordon Bleu

- **Snack:** Mini Pineapple Muffins

Day 24:

- **Breakfast:** Veggie And Hummus Wrap
- **Lunch:** Bean and Tuna Salad with White Balsamic Vinegar
- **Dinner:** Gingered Salmon Croquettes
- **Snack:** Almond Stuffed Prunes in Chocolate

Day 25:

- **Breakfast:** Whole Grain Waffles with Berry Compote
- **Lunch:** Scrambled Eggs with Dates
- **Dinner:** Beetroot Soup with Prune Dumplings
- **Snack:** Black Bean Brownies

Day 26:

- **Breakfast:** Ham and Cheese Croissant
- **Lunch:** Turkey-Roquefort Salad
- **Dinner:** Picadillo
- **Snack:** Red Marvel Smoothie

Day 27:

- **Breakfast:** Banana Oat Pancakes
- **Lunch:** Grilled Pesto Pizza
- **Dinner:** Quiche Lorraine
- **Snack:** Raspberry Lemon Cake

Day 28:

- **Breakfast:** Tofu Scramble
- **Lunch:** Chicken and Vegetable Stir-Fry
- **Dinner:** Asparagus Gratin with Spring Leeks
- **Snack:** Mini Pineapple Muffins

Day 29:

- **Breakfast:** Ricotta and Honey Toast
- **Lunch:** Bison Burgers with Sweet Potato Fries
- **Dinner:** Cod with Tomatoes and Black Olives
- **Snack:** Black Bean Brownies

Day 30:

- **Breakfast:** Greek Yogurt Parfait

- **Lunch:** Thick Frittata with Zucchini

- **Dinner:** Veal Cordon Bleu

- **Snack:** Almond Stuffed Prunes in Chocolate

CHAPER 4

Conclusion

In concluding this Osteoporosis Diet Cookbook for Seniors, it's essential to reflect on the transformative journey we've embarked upon together.

Nourishing our bodies is not merely a daily ritual; it's a conscious choice to embrace health and vitality, especially during the golden years.

The principles outlined in this cookbook are not just guidelines; they are pathways to better bone health, improved overall well-being, and a celebration of the joy that comes with savoring nutritious and flavorful meals.

Throughout these pages, we've delved into the intricacies of crafting a diet tailored for osteoporosis prevention and management.

From understanding the principles that underscore this diet to exploring a plethora of delectable recipes, our journey has been one of discovery and empowerment.

We've learned that food can be not only medicine for our bones but also a source of culinary delight.

The benefits of the Osteoporosis Diet extend beyond the physical realm. By embracing nutrient-rich foods and making informed choices, we empower ourselves to take charge of our health.

We've uncovered the importance of incorporating calcium, vitamin D, and other essential nutrients into our meals, recognizing that each bite is an investment in a stronger, more resilient tomorrow.

Armed with a comprehensive shopping list, a diverse array of recipes for every meal, and a 30-day meal plan for practical implementation, this cookbook serves as a compass guiding us towards a lifestyle that promotes bone health without sacrificing flavor.

It's not just a collection of recipes; it's a holistic approach to nurturing our bodies and minds.

As we close this chapter, let us carry forward the knowledge gained and the flavors experienced. Let this cookbook be a companion in the kitchen, a source of inspiration, and a reminder that every bite is an opportunity to fortify our bones and savor the richness of life.

May your culinary adventures continue, leading you to a path of health, happiness, and delicious discoveries. Cheers to vibrant living and the joy of savoring meals crafted with care!